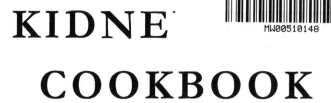

KIDNE

COOKBOOK

DELICIOUS LOW SODIUM KIDNEY-FRIENDLY RECIPES FOR RENAL HEALTH.

Mark D. Low

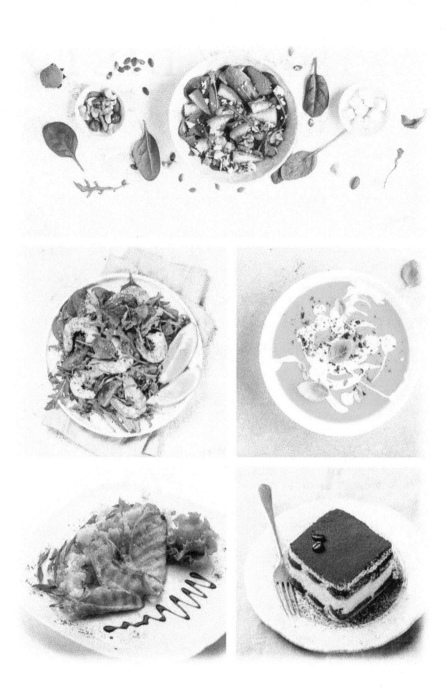

—

TABLE OF CONTENTS

Introduction _____ 7

Chapter 1 Breakfast _____ 10

   Sour Cream and Apple Bread _____ 12

   Vegetarian Rolls _____ 14

   Parmesan Zucchini Frittata _____ 16

   Crunchy Potato Croquettes _____ 18

   Zucchini Bread _____ 20

   Lemon and Broccoli Platter _____ 22

Chapter 2 Soups _____ 25

   Mediterranean Vegetable Soup _____ 27

   Tofu and Zucchini Soup _____ 29

   Bacon Cheeseburger Soup _____ 31

   Paprika Pork Soup _____ 33

   Onion Soup _____ 34

   Pan-Fried White Fish Soup _____ 36

Chapter 3 Poultry and Meat Mains _____ 39

   Chicken with Mushroom Sauce _____ 41

   Basil Lemon Turkey _____ 43

   Chicken in Herb Sauce _____ 44

   Beef chorizo _____ 46

   Beef and Three Pepper Stew _____ 47

   Spicy Lamb Curry _____ 48

Chapter 4 Seafood mains _____ 51

   Herbed Shrimps _____ 53

Sardine Fish Cakes_____55

Cajun Catfish _____57

Sage Salmon Fillet _____59

Fish Shakshuka_____61

Garlic Flavored Cod _____63

Chapter 5 Vegetarian Mains_____65

Delicious Vegetarian Lasagna_____67

Curried Cauliflower _____69

Chinese Tempeh Stir Fry_____71

Broccoli with Garlic Butter and Almonds _____72

Veg Stew _____74

Broccoli Steaks _____76

Chapter 6 Seasoning and Sauces _____79

Edamame Guacamole _____81

Herb Seasoning _____83

Basil Pesto Sauce _____85

Pepper and Lemon Seasoning_____87

Chicken and Turkey Seasoning _____88

Tzatziki Sauce _____90

Chapter 7 Desserts _____93

Frozen Lemon Dessert_____95

Italian Tiramisu Cheesecake_____97

Blueberry Peach Crisp _____99

Gingersnap Cookies _____101

Sweet Cracker Pie Crust_____103

Berry Ice Cream _____105

Bread Pudding _____107

Introduction

Healthy kidneys mean a healthy body. Kidneys help cleanse your body, eliminate toxins, and maintain the blood's biochemical balance.

The foods you consume are essential in managing your kidney health. If you are affected by kidney stones or CKD (Chronic Kidney Disease), you should control your intake of nutrients such as **protein, sodium, potassium, and phosphorus**.

Depending on the disease's stage and the patient's physical characteristics, these substances' tolerated levels may vary.
It is essential to control the amount of these substances in the food you eat each day to prevent CKD's worsening.

Preparing your own meals is an excellent strategy to improve the quality of the nutrients you take in, and consequently, it will help enhance your overall health.

Changing eating habits is strategic but can be challenging even if you know what you can or cannot eat. Having a variety of healthy and tasty recipes to build your new eating plan can make this change easier.

In this book, you will find clean and tasty recipes with correct protein, sodium, potassium, and phosphorus amounts to keep your kidneys healthy while satisfying your senses.

You can vary your meals every day and even indulge in a treat from time to time.

Kidney-friendly vegetables and fruits

Cabbage, green/red	Apples
Carrots	Cranberries
Cauliflower	Blackberries
Corn	Cherries
Cucumber	Grapefruit
Eggplant	Grapes
Celery	Figs, fresh
Chiles	Fruit cocktail
Chives	Macadamia Nuts
Arugula	Pears, canned
Asparagus	Pineapple
Bean sprouts	Lemon
Beets, canned	Lime
Ginger root	Peaches
Radishes	Plums
Vegetables, mixed	Tangerines
Green beans	Raspberries
Lettuce	Strawberries
Onions	Watermelon

Chapter 1
Breakfast

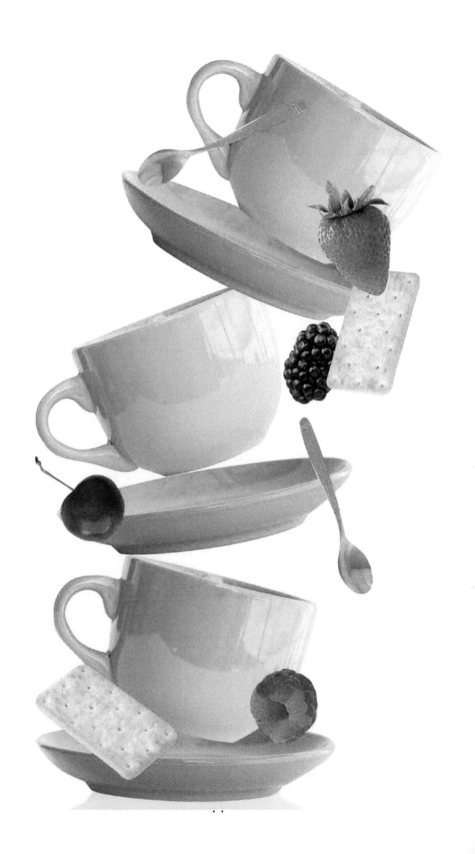

Preparation Time: 75 minutes

Servings: 4

Ingredients:
- 1 cup diced apple
- 1 ¾ cups all-purpose white flour
- ¾ teaspoon baking powder
- ½ cup white sugar
- ¼ teaspoon baking soda
- ½ teaspoon ground cinnamon
- ¼ cup canola oil
- 2 egg whites
- ¾ cup applesauce, unsweetened
- ¾ cup sour cream, reduced-fat
- 6 tablespoons water

Directions:
1. Preheat oven to 350°F.
2. Meanwhile, take a large bowl, add flour to it and then stir in baking soda and powder and cinnamon until mixed.
3. Take a separate bowl, add oil in it, beat in sugar until well combined, then gradually beat in flour mixture, egg whites, and applesauce until incorporated and fold in apples and sour cream until just mixed. Take an 8.5-by-4.75 inches loaf pan, grease it with oil, pour the batter in it and then bake for 55 minutes until the top has turned golden-brown and the loaf

passes the skewer test (if the skewer comes out clean from the center of the bread).

4. When done, let the loaf cool in the pan for 10 minutes, then take it out from the pan, and cool them for 20 minutes on the wire rack.

5. Cut the loaf into ten slices, and then serve.

Nutrition Facts per Serving:
Calories: 330 kcals, **Carbohydrates:** 49g, **Protein:** 6g, **Fat:** 12g, **Sodium:** 190mg, **Potassium:** 129mg, **Phosphorus:** 81mg

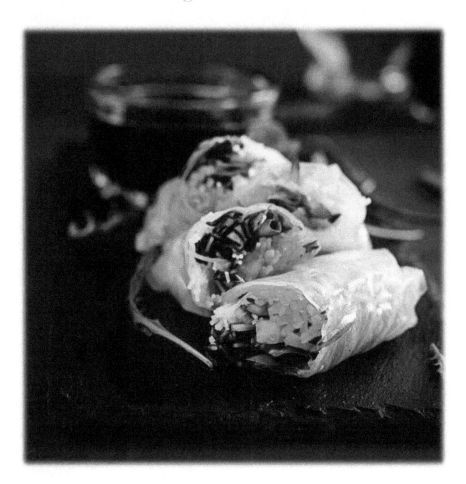

Preparation Time: 25 minutes
Servings: 4

Ingredients:

- 1-ounce rice vermicelli noodles
- 2 zucchinis shredded
- 2 carrots shredded
- 2 shallots finely chopped

- 2 small cucumbers peeled and diced
- ¾ cup fresh basil chopped
- ½ cup fresh cilantro chopped
- 12 spring roll wrappers

-

Dipping Sauce:
- 2 tablespoons honey
- 1/4 cup rice vinegar

2   fresh   red   chilies

-

Directions:
1. Place honey, vinegar, and 2 tablespoons of water in a saucepan and boil gently.
2. Remove from heat, add chilies, and set aside.
3. In a large bowl, combine all the ingredients (except wrappers).
4. Place a moistened wrapper on a work surface.
5. Put a spoonful of filling in the center and fold to encase, bringing corner to corner.
6. Fold in sides and roll up tightly. Brush end with water to seal.
7. Repeat until all filling is used.
8. Serve with dipping sauce.

Nutrition Facts per Serving:
Calories: 204 kcals, **Carbohydrates:** 45g, **Protein:** 6g, **Fat:** 1g, **Sodium:** 212mg, **Potassium:** 665mg, **Phosphorus:** 126mg

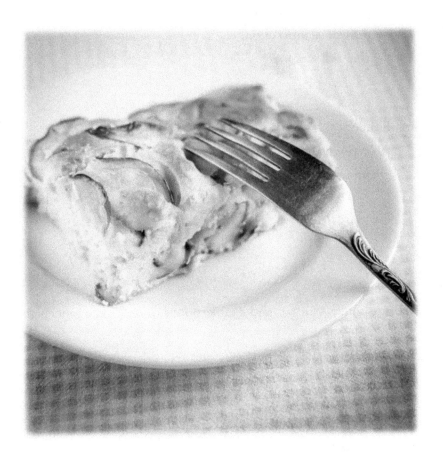

Preparation Time: 35 minutes
Servings: 4

Ingredients:

- 1 tablespoon olive oil
- 1 cup yellow onion, sliced
- 3 cups zucchini, chopped
- 2 tablespoons Parmesan cheese, grated
- 2 large eggs
- ½ cup milk, skimmed

- ½ teaspoon black pepper
- ⅛ teaspoon paprika

Directions:
1. Preheat the oven to 350°F.
2. Grease a 11x7 inches baking tray with cooking spray.
3. In a large bowl add eggs, milk, parmesan and stir well.
4. Add zucchinis, onion, paprika, pepper and stir gently.
5. Pour this mixture into the baking tray and spread it evenly.
6. Bake the zucchini casserole for approximately 20 minutes.
7. Cut in 4 slices and serve..

Nutrition Facts per Serving:
Calories: 74 kcals, **Carbohydrates**: 8g, **Protein:** 5g, **Fat:** 3g, **Sodium:** 53mg, **Potassium:** 390mg, **Phosphorus:** 122mg

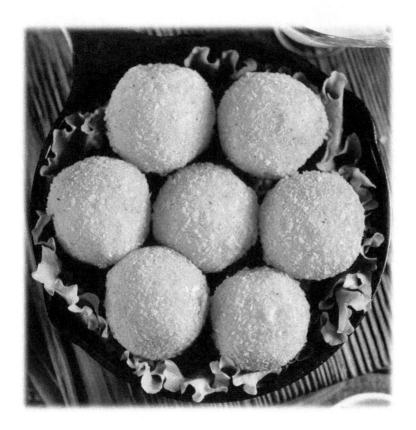

Preparation Time: 35 minutes

Servings: 4

Ingredients:
- 4 medium "leached" potato, cooked and peeled
- 1 tablespoon butter
- 1 tablespoon rice milk

- 1 tablespoon pepper
- 1 beaten egg
- 1 cup white breadcrumbs
- 2 tablespoon canola oil

Directions:
1. Mash potatoes with milk, butter, and pepper.
2. Form cooled potatoes into balls with your hands.
3. Dip balls in beaten egg.
4. Next, roll balls in breadcrumbs.
5. Then place balls in a hot oiled skillet and fry until golden brown.

Nutrition Facts per Serving:
Calories: 460 kcal, **Carbohydrates:** 73,33 g, **Protein:** 12 g, **Fat:** 13 g, **Sodium:** 381 mg, **Potassium:** 1039 mg, **Phosphorus:** 228 mg

Preparation Time: 1 hour 20 minutes
Cooking Time: 60 minutes
Servings: 6

Ingredients:
- 3 cups zucchini, grated
  2 cups all-purpose white flour
- 1 teaspoon herb seasoning (see recipe)
- 1 ½ teaspoons baking soda
- ¼ cup Splenda® granulated sweetener
- 1 ½ teaspoons pumpkin pie spice
- 2 tablespoons lemon juice
- 1 teaspoon vanilla extract, unsweetened
- 3 tablespoons honey
- 4 tablespoons olive oil
- 4 eggs
- ¾ cup applesauce, unsweetened

Directions:
1. Preheat the oven to 350°F.
2. Meanwhile, take a large bowl, add flour to it and then stir in herb seasoning (see recipe), Splenda®, baking soda, and pumpkin pie spice until mixed.
3. Take a separate bowl, crack eggs in it, beat until blended, stir in remaining ingredients until incorporated, and then stir this mixture gradually into flour mixture until combined. Don't over-mix.

4. Take two 8.5-by-4.5 inches loaf pans, distribute the batter evenly between them, and then bake for 60 minutes until the top has turned golden-brown, and loaves pass the skewer test (if the skewer comes out clean from the center of the bread).
5. When done, let the loaves cool in the pan for 10 minutes, take them out from the pan, and cool them for an additional 20 minutes on the wire rack.
6. Cut each loaf into twelve slices, and then serve.

Nutrition Facts per Serving:
Calories: 321 kcals, **Carbohydrates:** 47g, **Protein:** 8g, **Fat:** 12g, **Sodium:** 78mg, **Potassium:** 326mg, **Phosphorus:** 151mg

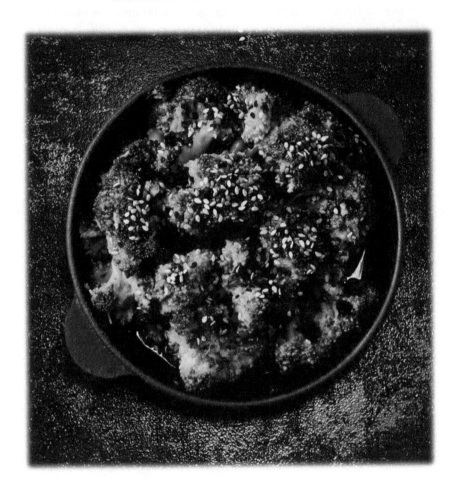

Preparation Time: 25 minutes
Servings: 4

Ingredients:
- 2 heads of broccoli, separated into florets
- 2 teaspoons extra virgin olive oil
- 1 teaspoon herb seasoning (see recipe)
- ½ teaspoon black pepper

- 1 garlic clove, minced
- ½ teaspoon lemon juice

Directions:
1. Preheat your oven to 400°F.
2. Bring a large pot of water to a boil and drop in the broccoli florets.
3. Boil the broccoli for 5 minutes. Remove, and drain.
4. Take a large-sized bowl and add broccoli florets.
5. Drizzle olive oil, season with pepper, herb seasoning, and garlic.
6. Spread the broccoli out in a single even layer on a baking sheet.
7. Bake for 15–20 minutes until fork tender.
8. Squeeze lemon juice on top.
9. Serve and enjoy!

Nutrition Facts per Serving:
Calories: 49 kcals, **Carbohydrates:** 6g, **Protein:** 3g, **Fat:** 3g, **Sodium:** 75mg, **Potassium:** 246mg, **Phosphorus:** 52mg

Chapter 2
Soups

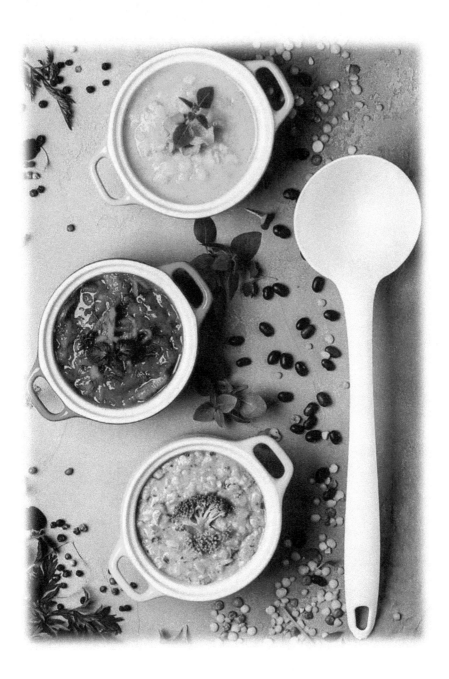

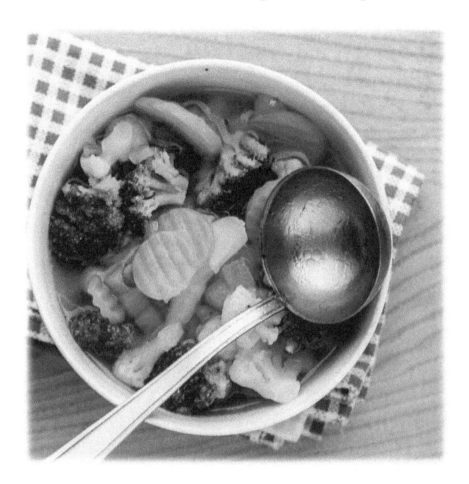

Preparation Time: 35 minutes
Servings: 4

Ingredients:

- 1 tablespoon extra-virgin olive oil
- 1 tablespoon oregano
- 2 minced garlic cloves
- 1 teaspoon black pepper

- 1 diced zucchini
- 1 cup diced eggplant
- 1 cup low sodium chicken stock
- 2 cups water
- 1 diced red pepper
- 1 diced red onion

Directions:
1. Soak the vegetables in warm water before use.
2. In a large cooking pot, add oil, chopped onion, and minced garlic.
3. Sauté for 5 minutes over medium heat.
4. Add the other vegetables to the onions and sauté for 8 minutes.
5. Add stock, water and bring to boil.
6. Stir in the herbs, reduce the heat, and simmer for a further 20 minutes.
7. Season with pepper to serve.

Nutrition Facts per Serving:
Calories: 70 kcals, **Carbohydrates:** 7g, **Protein:** 2g, **Fat:** 4g, **Sodium:** 44mg, **Potassium:** 321mg, **Phosphorus:** 44mg.

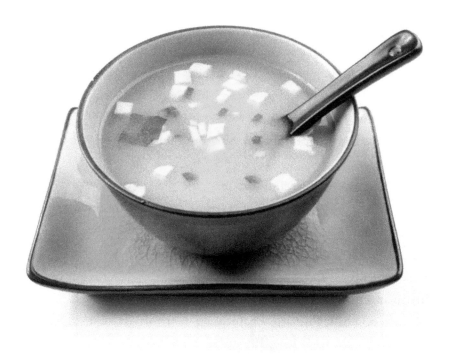

Preparation Time: 25 minutes
Servings: 2

Ingredients:

- 1 tablespoon miso paste
- 1/4 cup soft tofu, cubed
- 1 green onion, chopped
- 1 cup zucchini, diced

- ¼ cup Shiitake mushrooms, sliced
- 1 cup glutamate free vegetable stock
- 2 cups water
- 1/2 tablespoon soy sauce

Directions:
1. Take a saucepan, pour the stock and the water into this pan, and boil on high heat. Reduce heat to medium and let this stock simmer. Add mushrooms and zucchini and cook for almost 10 minutes.
2. Take a bowl and mix Soy sauce and miso paste together in this bowl.
3. Add this mixture and tofu in stock.
4. Simmer for nearly 5 minutes and serve with chopped green onion.

Nutrition Facts per Serving:
Calories: 33 kcals, **Fat:** 1 g, **Protein:** 4g, **Carbohydrates:** 4g, **Sodium:** 449mg, **Potassium:** 171mg, **Phosphorus:** 53mg

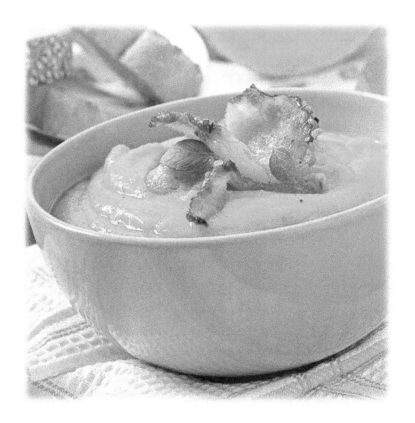

Preparation Time: 60 minutes
Servings: 2

Ingredients:

- 2 slices bacon
- 6 ounces ground beef
- 1 cup beef broth
- 1 cup water

- ½ teaspoon garlic powder
- ½ teaspoon onion powder
- 2 teaspoons brown mustard
- ½ teaspoon black pepper
- ½ teaspoon red pepper flakes
- 1 teaspoon cumin
- 1 teaspoon chili powder
- 1 medium dill pickle, diced
- ½ cup shredded cheddar cheese

Directions:

1. Start cooking the bacon in a non-stick pan until crispy, and then set aside.
2. Add ground beef in the bacon fat and cook over medium heat for 5 minutes, until browned on both sides.
3. Place beef in a cooking pot, add spices, and stir well.
4. Add broth, water, dill pickle, cheese, and stir until combined.
5. Simmer for 20 minutes over low heat, stirring occasionally.
6. Serve warm or hot with crispy bacon on top.

Nutrition Facts per Serving:

Calories: 339 kcals, **Carbohydrates:** 3g, **Protein:** 14g, **Fat:** 19g, **Sodium:** 286mg, **Potassium:** 275mg, **Phosphorus:** 181mg

Preparation Time: 40 minutes
Servings: 2

Ingredients:
- 4 oz. sliced pork loin
- 1 onion, diced
- 2 minced garlic cloves
- 1 cup baby spinach
- 3 cups water
- 1 tbsp. extra-virgin olive oil
- 1 tablespoon paprika
- 1 teaspoon black pepper

Directions:
1. In a large cooking pot, add the oil, chopped onion, and minced garlic.
2. Sauté for 5 minutes on low heat.
3. Add the pork slices to the onions and cook for 5 minutes or until browned.
4. Add paprika and water to the pan. Bring to a boil on high heat.
5. Stir in the spinach, reduce heat and simmer for 20 minutes
6. Season with pepper to serve.

Nutrition Facts per Serving:
Calories: 90 kcals, **Protein:** 7g, **Carbohydrates:** 5g, **Fat:** 5g, **Sodium:** 26mg, **Potassium:** 242mg, **Phosphorus:** 84mg.

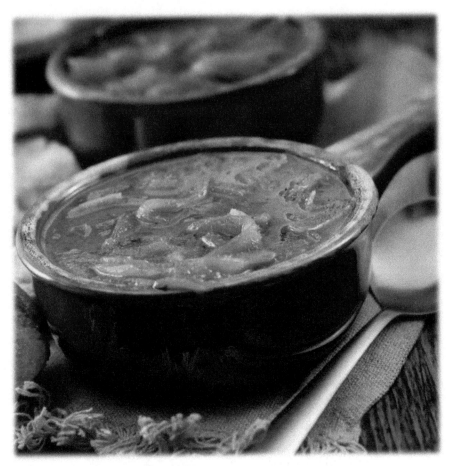

Preparation Time: 45minutes

Servings: 4

Ingredients:

- ½ cup chopped shiitake mushrooms
- 1 tablespoon grated ginger root
- 1 carrot, chopped
- 3 onions, diced
- ½ celery stalk, sliced

- ¼ tablespoon minced garlic
- 1 tablespoon butter
- 1 tablespoon minced chives
- 3 tablespoons beef bouillon
- 2 tablespoons chicken stock
- 2 cups water

Directions:

- In a non-stick cooking pot, combine butter, carrot, onions, celery, garlic, mushrooms and ginger.
- Sauté for 5 minutes.
- Add water, beef bouillon and chicken stock. Cook over high heat and let it boil.
- Decrease over medium heat and cover. Simmer for 20 minutes.
- Serve delicious soup in small bowls and sprinkle chives over each bowl.

Nutrition Facts per Serving:
Calories: 79 Kcals, **Carbohydrates:** 12g, **Protein:** 2g, **Fat:** 3g, **Sodium:** 67mg, **Potassium:** 285mg, **Phosphorus:** 64mg

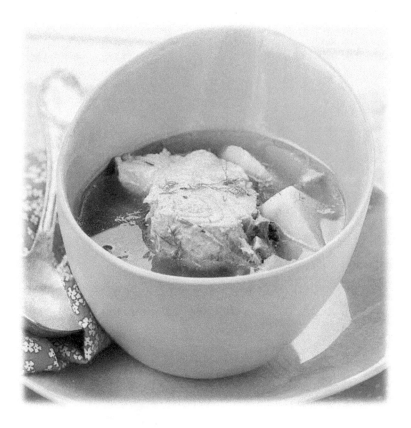

Preparation Time: 35 minutes

Servings: 4

Ingredients:

- 2 tablespoons olive oil
- 1 lb white fish, cubed
- 1 cup low-sodium vegetable stock
- ½ cup chopped onions
- 3 cups mixed vegetables
- ½ cup fresh chives, chopped

- 2 teaspoons herbal seasoning (see recipe)

Directions:
1. Sauté fish with olive oil in a large deep cooking pot for 3 minutes.
2. Add the seasoning, stock, and mixed vegetables.
3. Bring to boil over high heat and reduce to medium-low heat.
4. Cover and simmer for 20 minutes.
5. Remove from heat and sprinkle with fresh chives.
6. Serve and enjoy.

Nutrition Facts per Serving:
Calories: 220 kcals, **Carbohydrates:** 7g, **Protein:** 22 g, **Fat:** 10g, **Sodium:** 114mg, **Potassium:** 475mg, **Phosphorus:** 247mg.

Chapter 3

Poultry and Meat Mains

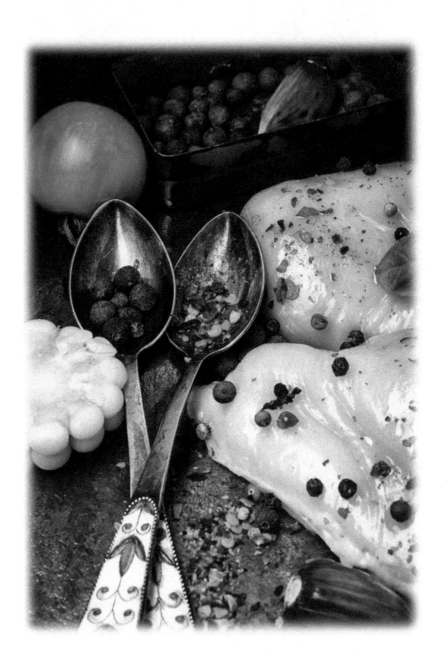

Preparation Time: 60 minutes
Servings: 4

Ingredients:
- 1 lb skinless chicken breast
- 1 cup mushrooms, sliced
- 2 bulbs of garlic
- 2 teaspoon herb seasoning
- ½ teaspoon dried thyme
- ¼ teaspoon ground black pepper
- ½ cup all-purpose white flour
- 4 teaspoons olive oil
- ½ cup skimmed milk
- 1 ½ cups chicken broth, low sodium

Directions:
1. Preheat the oven to 350°F.
2. Cut the top from each bulb of garlic, place bulb on a large piece of foil, cut-side up, drizzle with oil, wrap bulbs tightly, and then bake for 45 minutes, or until tender.
3. Meanwhile, wrap each chicken breast in a plastic wrap, and then pound with a meat mallet until ¼-inch thick.
4. Place flour in a shallow dish, stir in salt, thyme, and black pepper until combined, reserve 3 tablespoons of this mixture, and use the remaining mixture to coat the chicken.
5. Then take a large non-stick frying pan over medium-high heat, add 2 tablespoons olive oil and chicken, cook for 8 minutes.

When done, transfer chicken to a plate, cover with foil to keep it warm and set aside until needed.

6. When the garlic has baked, cool garlic bulbs for 10 minutes, gently squeeze the cloves, chop the garlic, and set aside

7. Add remaining oil in a skillet pan with mushrooms, cook for 5 minutes, or golden brown.

8. Sprinkle the reserved flour mixture over mushrooms, stir, cook for 2 minutes, add garlic, pour in milk and broth, stir until well combined, and bring the mixture to a boil.

9. Switch to low heat, simmer the mushroom sauce for 3 minutes until the sauce has thickened slightly, add chicken and coat it with the sauce—Cook for 2 more minutes.

10. Serve straight away.

Nutrition Facts per Serving:
Calories: 287 kcals, **Carbohydrates:** 21g, **Protein:** 31g, **Fat:** 8g, **Sodium:** 477mg, **Potassium:** 679mg, **Phosphorus:** 355mg,

Preparation Time: 10 minutes
Cooking Time: 25 minutes
Servings: 4

Ingredients:

- 1 pound turkey breast, sliced
- 4 teaspoons unsalted butter
- 1 cup water
- 1/4 cup fresh basil, minced
- 1/4 teaspoon garlic powder
- 1/4 teaspoon oregano
- 2 tablespoons lemon zest, grated

Directions:

1. Preheat oven to 325°F.
2. In a small ball, combine basil, garlic, oregano, and lemon zest.
3. Place the sliced breast in a roasting pan and add a hot water cup.
4. Pour spice mixture evenly over turkey breasts, making sure it is smoothly distributed. Pierce the turkey with a fork several times to allow the mixture to season and flavor as it cooks.
5. Add 1 teaspoon of butter on top of each slice.
6. Bake uncovered for 25 minutes or until juices in the turkey are clear, not pink.

Nutrition Facts per Serving:
Calories: 167 kcals, **Carbohydrates:** 1g, **Protein:** 27g, **Fat:** 5g, **Sodium:** 129mg, **Potassium:** 323mg, **Phosphorus:** 237mg

Preparation Time: 80 minutes

Servings: 2

Ingredients:
- 2 skinless chicken breasts
- ½ teaspoon garlic powder
- ¼ teaspoon celery salt
- ¼ teaspoon ground black pepper
- ½ teaspoon paprika
- ¼ teaspoon celery seeds
- ½ teaspoon mustard powder
- 3 tablespoons lemon juice
- 2 tablespoons butter, unsalted
- 1 tablespoon parmesan cheese, grated

-

Directions:
1. Preheat the oven to 350°F.
2. Take a small saucepan, place it over medium heat, add butter and when it melts, add all the ingredients (except for chicken and cheese), stir until mixed, and cook the sauce for 1 minute until hot.
3. Remove pan from heat, and then stir in cheese until it melts.

4. Take a baking dish, place chicken breasts in it, toss to coat with prepared sauce, and then bake for 30 minutes until the chicken is thoroughly cooked.

5. Serve hot.

Nutrition Facts per Serving:
Calories: 230 kcals, **Carbohydrates:** 2g, **Protein:** 32g, **Fat:** 10g
Sodium: 169mg, **Potassium:** 502 mg, **Phosphorus:** 317mg.

Preparation time: 20 minutes

Servings: 4

Ingredients:

- 3 garlic cloves, minced
- 1 lb. 90% lean ground beef
- 2 tbsp. hot chili powder
- 2 tsp. red or cayenne pepper
- 1 tsp. black pepper
- 1 tsp. ground oregano
- 2 tsp. white vinegar

Directions:

1. Mix all ingredients together in a bowl thoroughly, then spread it in a baking pan.
2. Bake the meat for 10 minutes at 325°F in the oven.
3. Slice and serve in crumbles.

Nutrition Facts per Serving: Calories: 72 kcals, **Protein:** 8g, **Carbohydrates:** 1g, **Fat:** 4g, **Sodium:** 46 mg, **Potassium:** 174 mg, **Phosphorus:** 79 mg

Preparation Time: 3 hours
Servings: 6

Ingredients:
- 12 ounces flat-cut beef brisket, whole
- 1 teaspoon dried thyme
- 1 teaspoon black pepper
- 1 garlic clove
- ½ cup green onion, thinly sliced
- 2 ½ cups water
- 1 tablespoon herb seasoning (see recipe)
- 1 large green bell pepper, sliced
- 1 large red bell pepper, sliced
- 1 large yellow bell pepper, sliced
- 1 large red onion, sliced

Directions:
1. In a large saucepan, put beef, spices, and water and sauté over medium heat.
2. Switch to low heat and for 2 hours, stirring every 20 minutes.
3. Add the sliced peppers and the onion.
4. Cook this over medium heat for 25 minutes until the vegetables are tender.
5. Serve hot and enjoy.

Nutrition Facts per Serving:
Calories: 252 kcals, **Carbohydrate:** 9g, **Protein:** 17g, **Fat:** 17g,
Sodium: 130 mg, **Potassium:** 520mg, **Phosphorous:** 188mg.

Preparation Time: 60 minutes

Servings: 6

Ingredients:
- 4 teaspoons ground coriander
- 4 teaspoons ground cumin
- ¾ teaspoon ground ginger
- 2 teaspoons ground cinnamon
- ½ teaspoon ground garlic cloves
- ½ teaspoon ground cardamom
- 2 tablespoons sweet paprika
- ½ tablespoon cayenne pepper
- 2 teaspoons chili powder
- 1-pound boneless lamb, trimmed and cubed into 1-inch size
- ground black pepper, to taste
- 1¼ cups water
- 1 cup coconut milk

Directions:
1. For spice mixture in a bowl, mix together all spices. Keep aside.
2. Season the lamb with black pepper.
3. In a large Dutch oven, heat oil on medium-high heat.
4. Add lamb and cook for approximately 4–5 minutes.
5. Stir in the spice mixture and cook for approximately 1 minute.
6. Add the remaining water and coconut milk and boil on high heat.

7. Reduce the heat to low and simmer, covered for approximately 40 minutes or until the lamb's desired doneness.

8. Serve hot.

Nutrition Facts per Serving:

Calories: 455 kcals, **Carbohydrate:** 11g, **Protein:** 23g, **Fat:** 36g, **Sodium:** 168mg,
Potassium: 611mg, **Phosphorous:** 271mg.

Chapter 4

Seafood mains

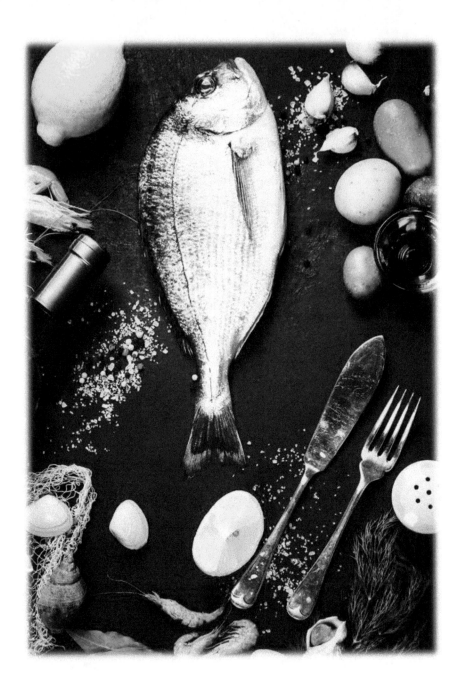

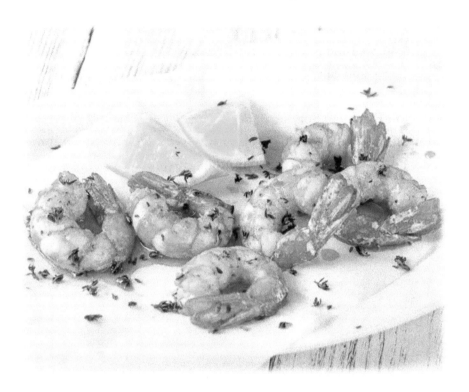

Preparation Time: 5 minutes
Servings: 4

Ingredients:

- 1/2 lb. shrimp, cooked, peeled, and deveined
- 1/2 cup reduced-fat sour cream
- 2 scallions, coarsely chopped
- 1 teaspoon lemon zest, finely grated
- 2 teaspoons fresh lemon juice

Directions:

1. Place the minced shrimp with the sour cream in a bowl.
2. Add in scallions, lemon juice, and lemon zest.
3. Mix well and refrigerate for 1 hour.
4. Serve and enjoy.

Nutrition Facts per Serving:

Calories: 97 kcals, **Carbohydrate:** 3g, **Protein:** 10g, **Fat:** 5g, **Sodium:** 86mg, **Potassium:** 235mg, **Phosphorous:** 137mg,

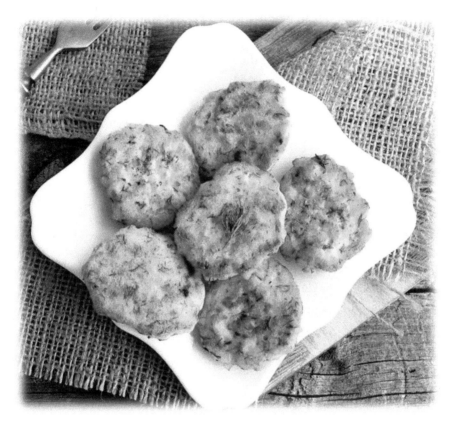

Preparation Time: 20 minutes
Servings: 4

Ingredients:

- 11 oz. sardines, canned, drained
- 1/3 cup shallot, chopped
- 1 teaspoon chili flakes
- 2 tablespoon wheat flour, whole grain
- 1 egg, beaten
- 1 teaspoon chives, chopped
- 1 teaspoon olive oil

- 1 teaspoon butter
-

Directions:
1. Put the butter in a non-stick frying pan and melt it.
2. Add shallot and cook it until translucent.
3. Transfer the shallot to the mixing bowl and add sardines, chili flakes, flour, egg, chives. Mix up until smooth with the help of the fork.
4. Make 8 medium size cakes and place them in the frying pan
5. Add olive oil.
6. Roast the fish cakes for 3 minutes from each side over medium heat.
7. Dry the cooked fish cakes with a paper towel if needed and transfer them to the serving plates.

Nutrition Facts per Serving:
Calories: 218 kcals, **Carbohydrate:** 5g, **Protein:** 21g, **Fat:** 12g, **Sodium:** 256mg, **Potassium:** 368mg, **Phosphorous:** 414mg.

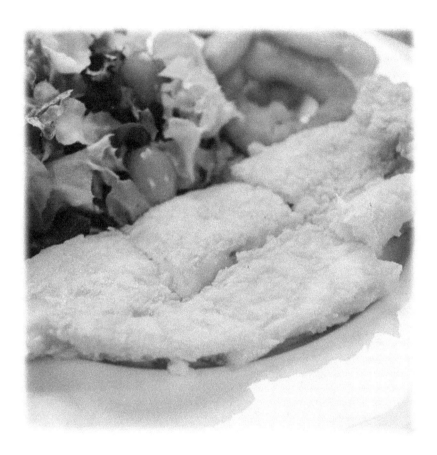

Preparation Time: 20 minutes
Servings: 4

Ingredients:

- 16 oz. catfish steaks (4 oz. each fish steak)
- 1 tablespoon Cajun spices
- 1 egg white, beaten
- 1 tablespoon sunflower oil

Directions:

1. Pour sunflower oil into a non-stick frying pan and preheat it.
2. Meanwhile, dip every catfish steak in the beaten egg and coat it in Cajun spices.
3. Place the fish steaks in the hot oil and roast them for 4 minutes from each side.
4. The cooked catfish steaks should have a light brown crust.
5. Serve and enjoy.

Nutrition Facts per Serving:
Calories: 176kcals, **Carbohydrate:** 1g, **Protein:** 18g, **Fat:** 10g, **Sodium:** 301mg, **Potassium:** 354mg, **Phosphorous:** 232mg.

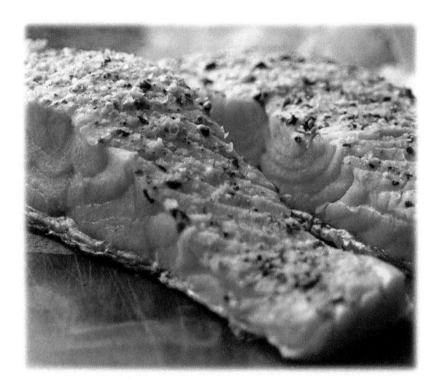

Preparation Time: 35 minutes

Servings: 4

Ingredients:

- 12 oz. salmon fillet
- 1 teaspoon sesame oil
- 1 tablespoon sage

Directions:

1. Rub the fillet with sage.
2. Place the fish in a baking tray and spray it with sesame oil.

3. Cook the fish for 30 minutes at 365°F.

4. Serve and enjoy

Nutrition Facts per Serving:

Calories: 165 kcals, **Carbohydrate:** 1g, **Protein:** 17g, **Fat:** 11g, **Sodium:** 41mg, **Potassium:** 314mg, **Phosphorous:** 177mg.

Preparation Time: 20 minutes

Servings: 4

Ingredients:

- 2 eggs
- 2 egg whites
- 1 cup tomatoes, chopped
- 3 bell peppers, chopped
- 1 tablespoon butter
- 1 teaspoon tomato paste
- 1 teaspoon chili pepper
- 1 tablespoon fresh dill
- 12 oz. cod fillet, chopped
- 1 tablespoon scallions, chopped
- ½ teaspoon black pepper

Directions:

1. Melt butter in a large non-stick frying pan.
2. Add chili pepper, bell peppers, and tomatoes.
3. Sprinkle the vegetables with scallions, dill, salt, and chili pepper. Sauté for 5 minutes.
4. Add chopped cod fillet and stir gently.
5. Close the lid and simmer the ingredients for 5 minutes over medium heat.
6. Slightly beat eggs and egg whites in a small bowl—season with black pepper.

7. Pour the beaten eggs over the fish and close the lid—Cook shakshuka with the closed lid for 5 minutes.

8. Serve and enjoy.

Nutrition Facts per Serving:
Calories: 163 kcals, **Carbohydrate:** 8g, **Protein:** 21g, **Fat:** 6g, **Sodium:** 130mg, **Potassium:** 375mg, **Phosphorous:** 83mg.

Preparation Time: 25 minutes
Servings: 4

Ingredients:
- 4 Cod fillets, 6 ounces each
- ¾ pound baby bok choy halved
- 4 tablespoons olive oil
- 2 tablespoon garlic, minced
- 1 teaspoon pepper

Directions:
1. Preheat your oven to 400°F.
2. Cut 3 sheets of aluminum foil (large enough to fit fillet).
3. Place cod fillet on each sheet and add oil and garlic on top.
4. Add bok choy, season with pepper.
5. Fold packet and enclose them in pouches.
6. Arrange on the baking sheet and bake for 20 minutes.
7. Let it cool for 10 minutes and serve.

Nutrition Facts per Serving:
Calories: 262 kcals, **Carbohydrates**: 4g, **Protein:** 28g, **Fat:** 15g,
Sodium: 197mg, **Potassium:** 8mg, **Phosphorus:** 1mg

Chapter 5

Vegetarian Mains

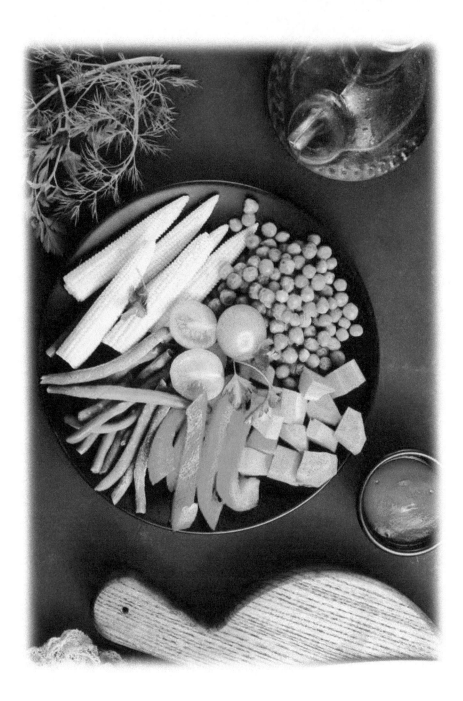

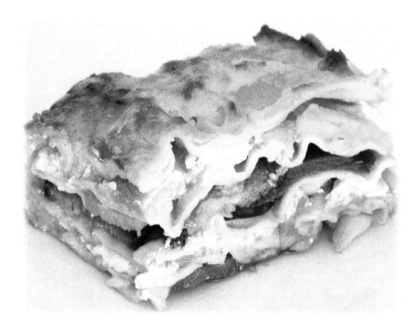

Preparation time: 70 minutes
Servings: 4

Ingredients:

- 1 teaspoon basil
- 1 tablespoon olive oil
- ½ red pepper, sliced
- 6 lasagna sheets
- ½ red onion, diced
- ¼ teaspoon black pepper
- 1 cup rice milk
- 1 garlic clove, minced
- 1 cup eggplant, sliced
- ½ zucchini, sliced
- 1 teaspoon oregano

Directions

- Preheat oven to 325°F/Gas Mark 3.
- Slice zucchini, eggplant and pepper into vertical strips.
- Add the rice milk and tofu to a food processor and blitz until smooth. Set aside.
- Heat the oil in a non-stick frying pan over medium heat. Add onion and garlic and sauté for 5 minutes.
- Sprinkle in the herbs, pepper, eggplant, zucchini and stir through for 10 minutes.
- Into a lasagna or suitable oven dish, layer 2 lasagna sheets, then 1/3 of vegetables.
- Repeat for the next 2 layers, finishing with the white sauce.
- Add to the oven for 50 minutes.
- Serve hot and enjoy.

-

Nutrition Facts per Serving:

Calories: 187 kcals, **Carbohydrates**: 32g, **Protein:** 5g, **Fat:** 5g, **Sodium:** 27mg, **Potassium:** 196mg, **Phosphorus:** 58mg

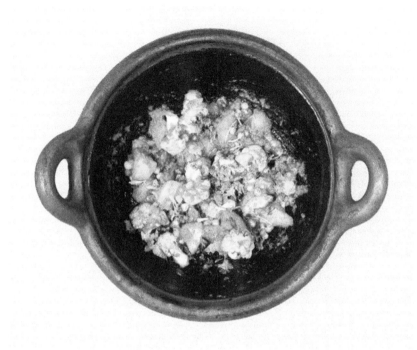

Preparation time: 25 minutes
Servings: 4

Ingredients:

- 1 teaspoon turmeric
- 1 onion, diced
- 1 tablespoon fresh cilantro. minced
- 1 teaspoon cumin
- ½ chili, minced
- ½ cup water
- 1 garlic clove, minced
- 1 tablespoon coconut oil

- 1 teaspoon curry
- 2 cups cauliflower florets

Directions

- Add the oil to a non-stick frying pan over medium heat.
- Sauté the onion and garlic for 5 minutes until soft.
- Add in cumin and turmeric and stir to release the aromas.
- Add chili to the pan along with the cauliflower.
- Stir to coat.
- Pour in the water and reduce the heat to a simmer for 15 minutes.
- Garnish with cilantro to serve.

Nutrition Facts per Serving:
Calories: 66 kcals, **Carbohydrates**: 7g, **Protein:** 2g, **Fat:** 19g, **Sodium:** 4 mg, **Potassium:** 20mg, **Phosphorus:** 222mg

Preparation time: 20 minutes

Servings: 2

Ingredients:

- 2 oz. tempeh, sliced
- 1 cup white rice, cooked
- 1 garlic clove, minced
- ½ cup green onions
- 1 tsp. minced fresh ginger
- 1 tbsp. coconut oil
- ½ cup corn

Direction:

- Heat the oil in a wok over high heat and add garlic and ginger.
- Sauté for 1 minute.
- Now add the tempeh and cook for 5-6 minutes before adding the corn for a further 10 minutes.
- Add the green onions and serve over white rice.

Nutrition Facts per Serving:
Calories: 120 kcals, **Carbohydrates**: 15g, **Protein:** 5g, **Fat:** 5g, **Sodium:** 105 mg, **Potassium:** 151mg, **Phosphorus:** 63mg

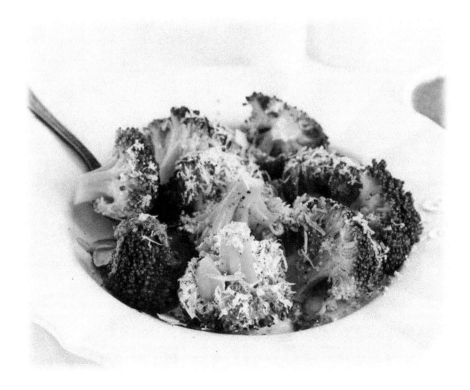

Preparation Time: 35 minutes

Servings: 3

Ingredients:

- 1 pound fresh broccoli, cut into bite-size pieces
- ¼ cup olive oil
- ½ tablespoon honey
- 1 tablespoon soy sauce
- ¼ teaspoon ground black pepper
- 2 cloves garlic, minced
- ¼ cup almonds, chopped

Directions:

1. Put broccoli into a large pot with about 1 inch of water in the bottom. Drain, and arrange broccoli on a serving platter.
2. Heat the oil in a small saucepan over medium heat—mix in the honey, soy sauce, pepper and garlic.
3. Bring to a boil, then remove from the heat.
4. Mix in the almonds and pour the sauce over the broccoli.
5. Serve immediately.

Nutrition Facts per Serving:

Calories: 220 kcals, **Carbohydrates**: 12g, **Protein:** 5g, **Fat:** 18g, **Sodium:** 268mg, **Potassium:** 425mg, **Phosphorus:** 116mg

Preparation time: 45 minutes

Servings: 4

Ingredients:

- 1 garlic cloves
- 1 cup white rice
- 1 teaspoon ground cumin
- 1 onion, diced
- 2 cups water
- 4 turnips, peeled and diced
- 1 teaspoon cayenne pepper
- ¼ cup chopped fresh parsley
- ½ teaspoon ground cinnamon
- 2 tablespoons olive oil
- 1 teaspoon ground ginger
- 2 carrots, peeled and diced

Direction:

1. In a large pot, heat the oil over medium heat and sauté onion for 5 minutes, until soft.
2. Add the turnips and sauté for 10 minutes.
3. Add garlic, cumin, ginger, cinnamon, and cayenne pepper, cooking for a further 3 minutes.
4. Add carrots and stock to the pot and then bring to a boil.
5. Switch to low heat and simmer for 20 minutes.

6. Meanwhile, add the rice to a pot of water and bring it to a boil.

7. Turn down to simmer for 15 minutes.

8. Drain and place the lid on for 5 minutes to steam.

9. Serve the vegetables on top of the rice and enjoy.

Nutrition Facts per Serving:

Calories: *297* kcals, **Carbohydrates**: 52*g*, **Protein:** 5g, **Fat:** 8g, **Sodium:** 112mg, **Potassium:** 474mg, **Phosphorus:** 113mg

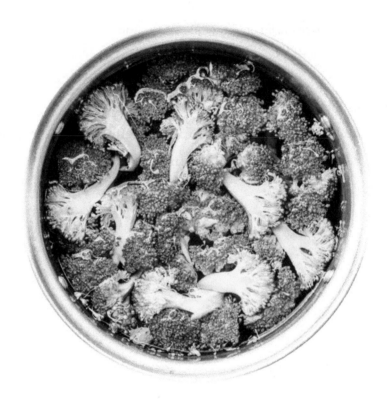

Preparation Time: 55 minutes

Servings: 2

Ingredients:

- 1 medium head broccoli
- 3 tablespoons olive oil
- ¼ teaspoon garlic powder
- ¼ teaspoon onion powder
- ¼ teaspoon pepper

Direction:

1. Preheat the oven to 400°F. Put parchment paper on a roasting pan.
2. Trim the leaves off the broccoli and cut off the stem's bottom. Cut the broccoli head in half. Cut each half into 1 to 3/4-inch slices, leaving the core in place. Cut off the smaller ends of the broccoli and save for another recipe. There should be 4 broccoli steaks.
3. Mix oil, garlic powder, onion powder, and pepper.
4. Lay the broccoli on the parchment-lined baking sheet.
5. Using half of the oil mixture, brush onto the broccoli—Bake for 20 minutes.
6. Remove from the oven and flip the steaks over.
7. Brush the steaks with remaining oil and roast for about 20 more minutes, until they are golden brown on the edges.
8. Serve hot or warm.

Nutrition Facts per Serving:
Calories: 109 kcals, **Carbohydrates**: 3g, **Protein:** 1g, **Fat:** 11g, **Sodium:** 13mg, **Potassium:** 125mg, **Phosphorus:** 26mg

Chapter 6

Seasoning and Sauces

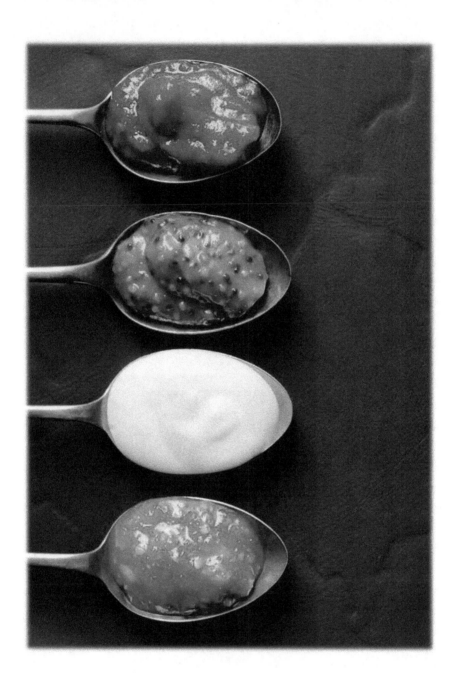

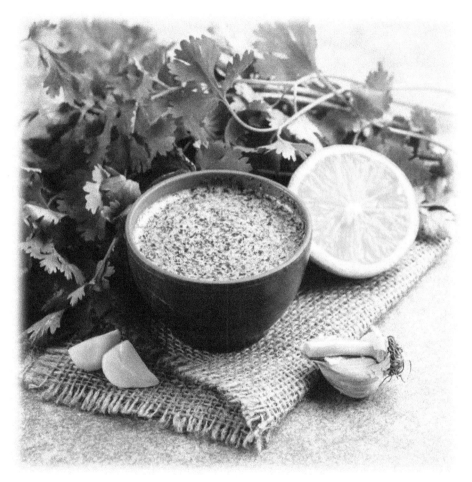

Preparation Time: 10 minutes
Servings: 4

Ingredients:

- 1 cup frozen shelled edamame, thawed
- ¼ cup water

- 1 lemon, juice and zest
- 2 tablespoons chopped fresh cilantro
- 1 tablespoon olive oil
- 1 teaspoon minced garlic

Directions:
1. In a food processor (or blender), add the edamame, water, lemon juice, lemon zest, cilantro, olive oil, and garlic, and pulse until blended but still a bit chunky.
2. Serve fresh.

Nutrition Facts per Serving:
Calories: 63 kcals, **Fat:** 5g, **Carbohydrates:** 12g, **Protein:** 3g, **Sodium:** 3mg, **Phosphorous:** 100mg, **Potassium:** 64mg

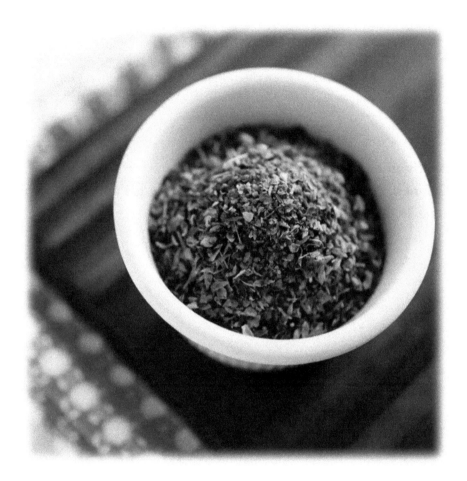

Preparation Time: 15 minutes

Servings: 6

Ingredients:

- 2 teaspoons dried garlic
- 2 teaspoons dried thyme
- 1 teaspoon paprika

- 1 teaspoon cinnamon
- 1 teaspoon dried basil
- 1 teaspoon dried ginger

Directions:

Mix all spices and keep them in an airtight container. Good for up to one year.

Nutrition Facts per Serving:
Calories: 5 kcals, **Carbohydrates:** 1 g, **Protein:** 1 g, **Fat:** 1 g, **Sodium:** 1 mg, **Potassium:** 19 mg, **Phosphorus:** 3 mg.

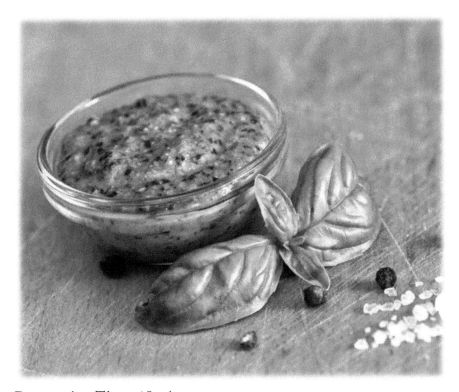

Preparation Time: 15 minutes
Servings: 4

Ingredients:

- 8 tablespoons olive oil
- 1 garlic clove
- 3 cups fresh basil leaves
- 1 tablespoon pine nuts
- 1 teaspoon Parmesan cheese

Directions:

1. Put all of the ingredients into a food processor and blend until smooth.

2. Store prepared pesto sauce in a jar or covered container until ready to use. Keep it for up to a week in the refrigerator.
3. Serve with pasta, pizza, salads.

Nutrition Facts per Serving:
Calories: 272 kcals, **Carbohydrates:** 1g, **Protein:** 1g, **Fat:** 30g, Sodium: 7mg, **Potassium:** 70 mg, **Phosphorus:** 14mg.

Preparation Time: 15 minutes
Servings: 4

Ingredients:

- 1 teaspoon ground coriander seeds
- 2 lemons
- 2 tablespoons cracked peppercorns

Directions:

1. Heat an oven to the lowest temperature setting. Wash and dry the lemons. Remove the yellow part of the lemon peel by finely grating it.
2. Mix the finely grated lemon zest with the cracked peppercorns.
3. Layout the mixture on a flat cooking sheet that has been lined. Put the flat cooking sheet in the oven for one hour and fifteen minutes, stirring mixture for a minimum of every twenty minutes.
4. Add the coriander to the mixture and place it into a food processor to finely grind.
5. Store it in an airtight container. It can be used to replace table salt.

Nutrition Facts per Serving:
Calories: 21 kcals, **Carbohydrates:** 6 g, **Protein:** 1 g, **Fat:** 1 g, **Sodium:** 2 mg, **Potassium:** 103 mg, **Phosphorus:** 13 mg

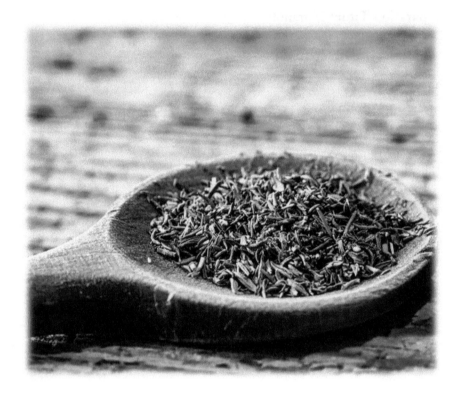

Preparation Time: 15 minutes
Servings: 6

Ingredients:

- 6 teaspoons sage
- 6 teaspoons thyme
- 1 teaspoon ground pepper
- 2 teaspoons dried marjoram

Directions:

Mix all spices and keep them in an airtight container. Good for up to one year.

Nutrition Facts per Serving:
Calories: 5 kcals, **Carbohydrates:** 1 g, **Protein:** 1 g, **Fat:** 1 g, **Sodium:** 1 mg, **Potassium:** 19 mg, **Phosphorus:** 3 mg.

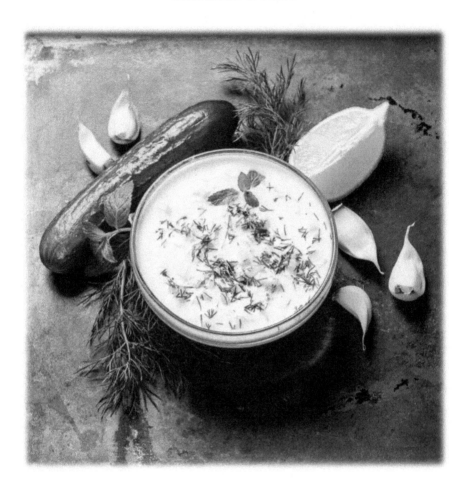

Preparation Time: 35 minutes
Servings: 4

Ingredients:

- cucumber, grated (2 cups)
- 1 cup 2% plain Greek yogurt
- 1 large clove garlic, minced
- 2 tablespoons extra-virgin olive oil

- 1 tablespoon lemon juice
- 1 tablespoon fresh dill, minced

Directions:
1. Place the grated cucumber in a fine-mesh strainer set over a bowl for 10 minutes.
2. Use a potato masher and press the cucumber to release the liquid. Repeat two more times for a total of 30 minutes.
3. While the cucumber is draining, combine the rest of the ingredients in a mixing bowl.
4. Incorporate the cucumber into the mixed ingredients.
5. Store refrigerated for up to 3 days.

Nutrition Facts per Serving:
Calories: 74 kcals, **Carbohydrates**: 6g, **Protein:** 3g, **Fat:** 8g, **Sodium:** 40mg, **Potassium:** 208mg, **Phosphorus:** 71mg.

Chapter 7

Desserts

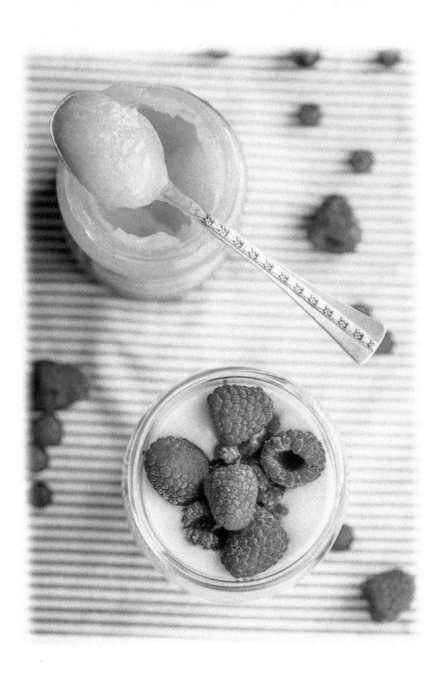

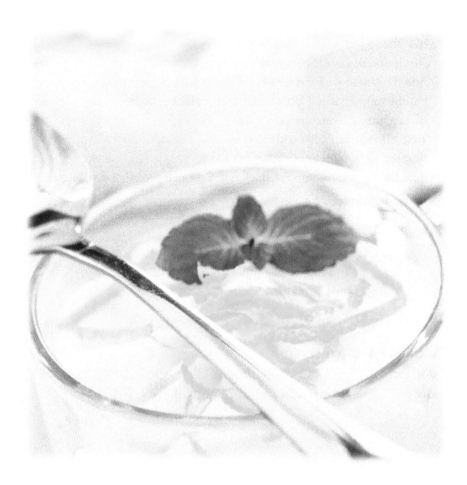

Preparation Time: 20 minutes
Servings: 2

Ingredients:
- 4 eggs, separated
- ¼ cup lemon juice
- 2/3 cup sugar
- 1 tablespoon lemon peel, grated
- 2 cups vanilla wafers, crushed

- 1 cup whipped cream

Directions:

1. Beat the egg yolks until they become very thick.
2. Slowly add sugar and beat each time you add.
3. Add the lemon peel and lemon juice, mix well.
4. Put the mixture in a double boiler and cook over boiling water, constantly stirring until the mixture gets thick.
5. Take off heat and keep aside to cool.
6. Beat the egg whites until stiff.
7. Pour the egg whites into the thick mixture once cooled. Add whipped cream and stir.
8. Spread one and a half crumbs of the vanilla wafer in the bottom of a baking dish or freezer tray.
9. Scoop the lemon mixture and spread over the crumbs.
10. Sprinkle the remaining vanilla wafer crumbs on the top.
11. Freeze for 5 hours until the mixture is firm.

Nutrition Facts per Serving:
Calories: 387 kcals, **Carbohydrates**: 44g, **Protein:** 6g, **Fat:** 22g, **Sodium:** 139mg, **Potassium:** 117mg, **Phosphorus:** 106mg

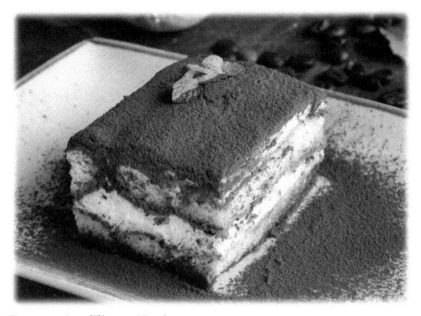

Preparation Time: 45 minutes

Servings: 10

Ingredients:

- 6 egg whites, whipped
- 10 ounces mascarpone cheese
- ½ cup sugar
- 1 teaspoon vanilla extract
- 4 ounces brewed espresso
- 1 tablespoon bitter cocoa powder

Directions:

1. Cut the pound cake into ten even slices, and set it aside
2. Mix the cheese, vanilla, and sugar in a bowl until it is smooth. Add the whipped eggs.
3. Pour the espresso into a shallow dish

4. Dip the sides of 4 pieces of pound cake into the espresso, placing them in an 8 –inch loaf pan. Break the pieces up, if required to coat the bottom of the pan
5. Gently spread ⅓ of the cream cheese mixture over the cake—repeat the procedure with the remaining slices of pound cake to make three layers.
6. Sprinkle cocoa powder on top.
7. Refrigerate for about 3 hours, then cut into pieces of 10 and serve

Nutrition Facts per Serving:
Calories: 174 kcals, **Carbohydrates:** 12g, **Protein:** 4g, **Fat:** 13g, **Sodium:** 53mg, **Potassium:** 105mg, **Phosphorus:** 24mg

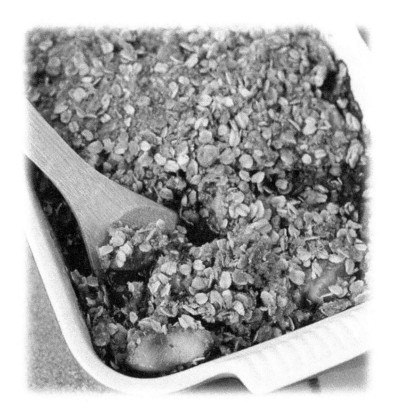

Preparation Time: 55 minutes
Servings: 6

Ingredients:
- 7 medium-sized fresh peaches
- 1 cup blueberries
- ¼ cup granulated sugar
- 1 tablespoon lemon juice
- ¾ cup all-purpose flour
- ¾ cup packed brown sugar

99

- ½ cup butter

Directions:
1. Preheat oven to 375°F
2. Pit and slice the peaches into ¾- inch slices
3. Use a cooking spray to spray a 12 x 9-inch baking dish, then place the peach slices and blueberries on top of the dish
4. Sprinkle over the fruit, sugar, and lemon juice
5. Use a small bowl to combine and mix the flour and brown sugar
6. Cut the butter into the flour mixture using two knives or a pastry blender until it is crumbly. Sprinkle the crumbs on top of the fruit
7. Bake for about 45 minutes or until the fruit becomes soft and the crumbs are browned, then serve warm.

Nutrition Facts per Serving:
Calories: 353 kcals, **Carbohydrates:** 54g, **Protein:** 3g, **Fat:** 15g, **Sodium:** 9mg, **Potassium:** 261mg, **Phosphorus:** 45mg

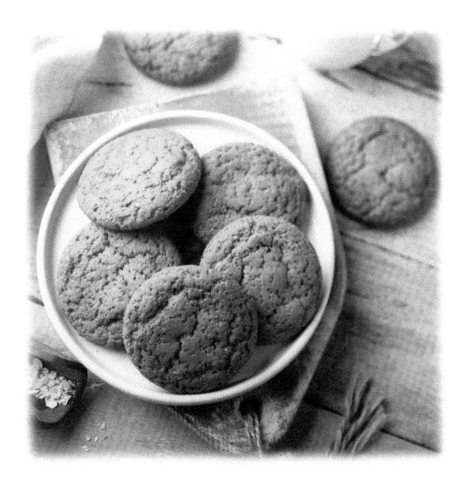

Preparation Time: 1 hour 20 minutes
Servings: 6

Ingredients:

- 2 cups all-purpose white flour
- 3 teaspoons baking soda
- 1 teaspoon ground ginger
- 1 teaspoon ground cinnamon

- 1 stick unsalted softened butter
- 1 cup granulated sugar
- 1 egg
- 2 tablespoons molasses

Directions:

1. Sift together the flour, baking soda, ginger and cinnamon
2. Cream the butter using a mixer until it becomes light and fluffy, add sugar gradually, then blend in the egg and molasses
3. Pour in a small amount of the flour mixture at a time until a dough is formed
4. Cover and store in the refrigerator for 1 hour or overnight
5. Preheat oven to 350°F
6. Form the dough into a heaped teaspoon ball size, and place 2-inch apart on top of a greased cookie sheet. Slightly flatten each ball.
7. Bake for about 8 to 10 minutes, then cool on a wire rack.
8. Serve and enjoy.

Nutrition Facts per Serving:
Calories: 450 kcals, **Carbohydrates**: 72g, **Protein:** 5g, **Fat:** 16g, **Sodium:** 18mg, **Potassium:** 316mg, **Phosphorus:** 170mg

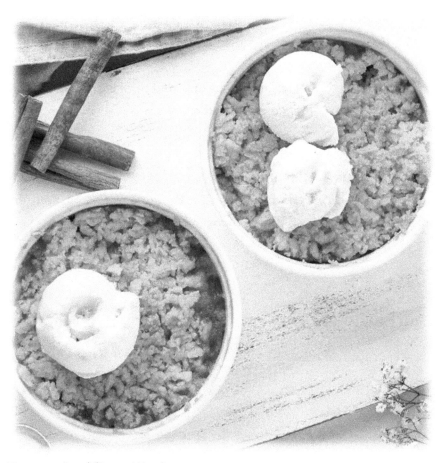

Preparation Time: 15 minutes

Cooking Time: 20 minutes

Servings: 2

Ingredients:

- 1 bowl gelatin cracker crumbs
- 1/4 small cup sugar
- 3 teaspoons unsalted butter
- ½ cup whipped cream

Directions:

1. Preheat the oven to 375°F.
2. Mix sweet cracker crumbs, butter, and sugar.
3. Put in a baking tray and then in the oven.
4. Bake for 7 minutes.
5. Let the pie cool before adding any kind of filling.
6. Serve with whipped cream and enjoy.

Nutrition Facts per Serving:
Calories: 184 kcals, **Carbohydrates**: 27g, **Protein:** 1g, **Fat:** 1g, **Sodium:** 2mg, **Potassium:** 24mg, **Phosphorus:** 15mg

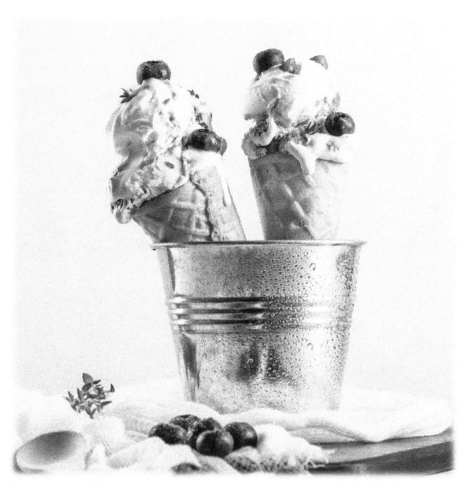

Preparation Time: 10 minutes
Servings: 6

Ingredients:

- 6 ice cream cones
- 1 cup whipped topping
- 1 cup fresh blueberries
- 4 oz. cream cheese

- 1/4 cup blueberry jam

Directions:
1. Put the cream cheese in a large cup and beat it with a mixer until it is fluffy.
2. Mix with fruit and jam and whipped topping.
3. Put the mixture on the small ice cream cones and refrigerate them in the freezer for 2 hours.
4. Serve and enjoy.

Nutrition Facts per Serving:
Calories: 177 kcals, **Carbohydrates:** 21g, **Protein:** 3g, **Fat:** 10g, **Sodium:** 91mg, **Potassium:** 72mg, **Phosphorus:** 43mg

Bread Pudding

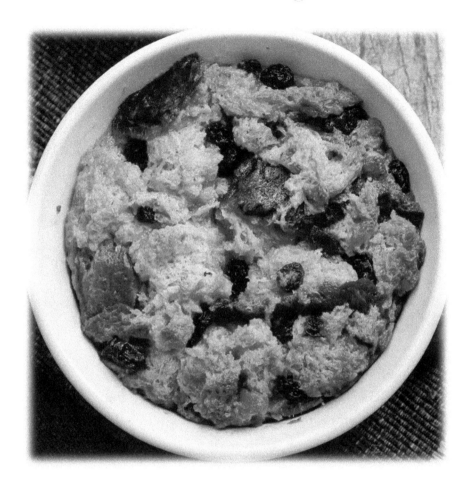

Preparation Time: 55 minutes
Servings: 6

Ingredients:

- 2 eggs
- 2 egg whites
- 1½ cups almond milk
- 2 tablespoons honey

- 1 teaspoon vanilla
- 2 tablespoons rum or 1 teaspoon rum extract
- 4 slices of raisin bread

Directions:

1. Preheat oven to 325° F
2. Use a non-stick cooking spray to spray an 8-inch round baking dish
3. Beat the eggs and egg white in a large mixing bowl until it is foamy. Beat in the almond milk, vanilla, honey, and the rum or rum extract
4. Cut the bread into cubes, stir into the egg mixture then spread over the baking dish
5. Bake for about 35 to 40 minutes or until it comes out clean when a knife is inserted at the center
6. Spoon out warm pudding into dishes to serve.

Nutrition Facts per Serving:
Calories: 105 kcals, **Carbohydrates:** 16g, **Protein:** *4g*, **Fat:** 2g, **Sodium:** 111mg, **Potassium:** 89mg, **Phosphorus:** 44mg